How To Keep Erect Naturally

K.B.

The Author provides the content contained therein for informational purposes only. The Author does not provide any medical advice in the book, and the Information should not be so construed or used. None of this content is to replace the services of a licensed, trained physician or health professional or to be a substitute for medical advice of a physician or trained health professional licensed in your state. You should not rely on anything contained in the book, and you should consult a physician licensed in your state in all matters relating to your health. You hereby agree that you shall not make any health or medical related decision based in whole or in part on anything contained in the book.

This is the full transcript of an interview with herbal genius Logan Christopher from November 2013 which has been released under The Bliss Show. The intentions of the show are to inform fans about the many natural alternatives for them on long lasting stamina.

The Bliss Show is a weekly program for men and women that reveals sexual freedom technologies proven and backed by science.

The host of the Bliss Show is none other than sex researcher and speaker Kali DuBois M.A. Human Sexuality, B.A. Human Development, C. hT.

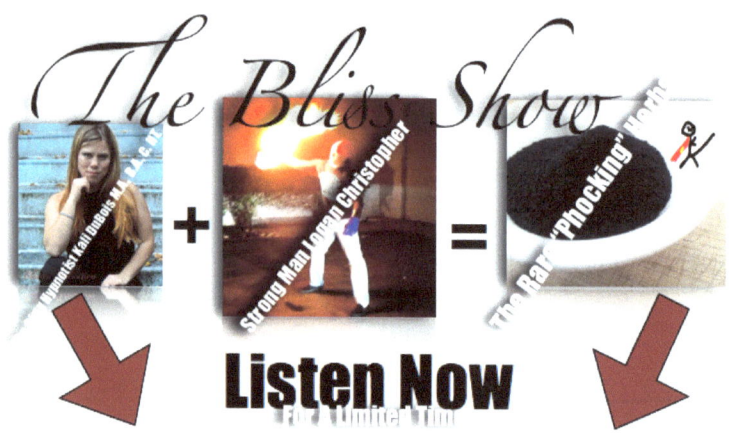

Listen to the live recording of this book

http://www.kaliblissshow.com/herbs

Recommended Resources

Sexual Energy Healing For Men:

http://www.EnergyViagra.com

Hypnosis For Sex:

http://www.HypnosisForSex.com

KALI: So today on the Bliss Show we have Logan Christopher, a strong man and herbal researcher. He's going to reveal herbs for peak performance, erection helping herbs, herbs to help increase testosterone, herbs that help with increasing penis growth, and so much more.

These are secret herbs because little is known about them in the West. These are herbs you can't just go out and buy at Whole Foods or a vitamin shop. These are herbs you can't find practically anywhere. I know because I went out looking for them locally, before I bought them from Logan seven months back.e.

I've tried a lot of his herbs to help with peak performance training in the martial arts. So to begin the show I want to introduce you guys to Logan Christopher.

Kali: Say hi Logan. Hi Logan!

Logan: Hello! Thanks for having me on the Bliss Show.

Kali: I've known you for a couple years. We met through martial arts. So can you tell my audience a synopsis about how you walks your talk, especially when it comes to herbs, male health and physical conditioning.

Logan: What led me into getting into researching these herbs is that I do a lot of strength training and fitness conditioning.

It's not your average strength training. I do things like bend horseshoes, rip phone books in half and a lot training with kettlebells, bodyweight exercise, backflips, and handstands.

I model after the old time Strong Men, having done feats like pulling a fire truck by my hair. So I just don't do the average things - I do things a little different than what most people are exposed to in a regular gym. My goals are to become as strong as I possibly can.

[In the 19th century, the term **strongman** referred to performers who did strength feats like card tearing, nail bending, supporting large amounts of weight held overhead at arm's length, steel bending, chain breaking, etc. Large amounts of wrist, hand, tendon strength are required for these feats.

Kali: Okay, so his goal is to become a strong as he possibly can.

I once saw you, Logan, bend a horseshoe and rip a stack of phone books. I went over your house one day when you moved up here to Oregon to train with Doc and you were showing me juggling kettle bells and I was just amazed. I don't know if you heard, but that horseshoe you bent into a heart was stolen off sports psychologist Dr. John La Tourrette's desk. I was like okay that's intense.

Logan: I had to bring him a replacement after that happened. It's not a problem I can bend lots of horseshoes.

Kali: Now for the first time listener, can you explain what peak performance is and what it means to you? I mean, I know you do a lot of strong man and a lot of different type of feats but what does peak performances mean to you?

Logan: Peak performance is not just about strength and fitness… That is sort of my direction because I have a lot of fun with it. But with peak performance is applicable to all areas. You can have peak performance for fitness. You can also have peak performance for your sex life. You can also have peak performance for everyday life:
when working, your business, your job, whatever it may be.

The idea of peak performance is to be able to perform at your best. To be at a high level all the time. I don't know about you but that is certainly something I want. I do not like going through the low points of life. I want to do everything I possibly can. And that is why I combine stuff like training and with lots of nutritional supplements in order to really be at my peak all the time, so I can accomplish all the things I want to do.

Kali: That is a good way of putting it. I definitely have trained in mind sciences and athleticism to stay on top. The same thing goes sexually. The reason I have you here is that you kind of practically stumbled upon the sexual effects of the peak performances by experimenting. Because you are the type of guy that tests everything and I know these personally because I have sparred with you. You are always experimenting, you are always looking for what works. I find it amazing to be able to discuss peak performance with you and go, "wow." And once you are on that top and you are doing everything the best you can, you start to find things bleed over into other areas of your life.

And peak performance sexually and that's what my listeners are all about. They always ask me, "why is it happening to me?"

"What is happening to me?" [Low erections, sexual problems].

Basically because they have dropped down and they are no longer performing at top level. There could be all different types of reasons. If we were going to really hyper-focus on the sexual effects of peak performance and the herbs and the training you've done we then can now go into the biology on why most people drop.

It could be because they are not working out. They are not taking the right nutrition into their body. They are not taking the herbs. I'm not talking about taking Viagra. Viagra is just fixing side effects. There is more to the whole way of living your life.

I want to go over the causes of these problems, how they are directly related to those three things, and the dropping down into a low area of their life and not being on top of their peak performance.

I am going to go into the biology of what can cause erection problems. I get emails from people who come from all different walks of life. All different age groups and they all have different desires for where they want to take their sex life.

I'm going to cover some of these first then we will go into how Logan defines peak performance and herbs and the sexual effects you stumbled upon.

Most erection problems are usually because a shortage of key hormone testosterone. This is a hormone that you can increase by being a strong man. By being an athlete.

Erection problems are also caused by fatigue, stress and low energy levels.

Erection problem can also be caused by poor blood circulation, which leads to not having enough blood pumped to the genitals.

A lack of nitric oxide also contributes to erection problems. Nitric Oxide is the key to getting an erection in the first place.

You probably know you need testosterone, you probably know low energy levels will kill your sex drive and peak performance and erection.

The body converts the amino acid L-arginine into nitric oxide. The FDA says a dose of 5 grams of L-Arginine increases a person's nitric oxide levels.
I know a few people who actually went out and tested how much L-Arginine they needed to take to have sexual effects. They needed a lot more than the 5 grams suggested by FDA - these people were actually taking up to 20 grams of L-Arginine a day for the sexual effects to occur. Because of the very high dose, yhey were having serious side effects like loose stools.

There are other things you can do instead of taking L-Argenine.

If you have erection problems the chances are you have very sluggish circulation. That is why a lot people seek tantric massage as a natural way to help increase circulation. The blood needs to arrive at the genital area to increase the volume for an erection to occur. When it gets there the blood needs to enter the lingam [Sanskrit for the penis]. This is where the nitric oxide plays its key role. It allows the blood vessels to relax and expand which feed the penis. When the vessels widen an increase flow of blood enters and the result is an erection.

That is the biology behind it and what can we do about the stress, having low nitric oxide, having poor circulation. Well we go to get you back to that peak performance level Logan Christopher is at constantly.

This guy is constantly intense because he is testing and he is experimenting with everything to find what works.

Logan walks his talk, and to do this he has developed a herbal line with his brothers.

KALI: What is it like behind the scenes? You experiment, your clients experiment and what has been reported back to you?

LOGAN: We are always experimenting like you said, that's something I do because in order to constantly pursue peak performance. It's not really you have peak performance or you don't, there are all sorts of different levels. Mine is trying push the level further. So I have been experimenting with my exercise and physical things that I do. I have been experimenting with my nutrition. Experimenting with my mindset.

When entering the whole thing there's always experimenting going on, and going beyond.

With these herbs it's very different. There's a whole bunch of different herbs out there and some are better than others. That is something I will be discussing. We've had some pretty phenomenal results in different areas and definitely lots of stories back from our customers. I'll be sharing some of those today.

KALI: Okay cool! You said there are several herbs you have tried. I know you've tried a lot because I've seen your pantry and I've seen the thousands of things you have in there. Like crazy things - it's like opening a mad scientist's closet and seeing 'eyeballs in jars'.

Logan, you try everything. One time when you came home from a convention on Chinese Medicine and you had all these mushrooms and I was like, "what are these?" And you said, "don't touch that!" I was shocked, "okay!"

I know my listeners are eager to know what these secrets herbs are, and what you suggest, what you have experimented with. So can you tell us about those herbs?

LOGAN: Yeah! Absolutely! Before going into the herbs I want to talk about herbalism just a little bit. When people hear the word herb-what they have in mind is something that many people use for medicine. For instance, if you're getting sick then taking echinacea can be good for boosting your immune system. And its not something you wanna be on all the time because that's what echinacea does, it boosts your immune system. So in the cases of immune disorders that's not something you necessary want to have.

In the Chinese Medicine system there is an 'inferior' class of herbs - 'inferior' in that they are not as great as the superior class of herbs.

The superior herbs are what I really focus much more on. With the superior class of herbs you have stuff that you can take long term. Some of these herbs you can take literally every single day for the rest of your life and it would not just support your health.

Most of these are adaptogens. This means they can boost your immune system when needed, and can also scale it back when its needed. They have intelligence when working with the body. These are unlike drugs where you have one specific chemical that's been isolated.

Many drugs originally came from plants, or different herbs. A specific chemical was isolated and amplified to where you have a thousand times of what the natural plant originally had. Some drugs are very useful for what they do, but most drugs also have undesired side effects.

The truth is side effects can only be called side effects if you notice them. What is really happening behind the scenes in your body when you take a drug is that it lowers your overall health in many different ways. You really only begin to notice side effects once they pass a threshold where they are noticeable.

So that's the difference between herbs and drugs. Also some herbs are not good when they are compared to other herbs. As I said earlier, I'm really focused on the superior class of herbs that have a much greater effect in boosting your health as well as achieving peak performance.

KALI: Wow! So there's classification. I have studied Chinese Medicine myself and I find it interesting how you focus directly on the superior class of adaptogens and how they work synergistically. Like you said, it's not like echinacea which is taken for a short period of time, like when you have cold. You can take these herbs over a long period of time because the effects are different for your level of health.

LOGAN: Yes. There is also the idea in Chinese Medicine on Radiant Health. That is having health beyond danger. You get to a point where you won't become sick at all. I can't remember the last time I got sick. This is because I'm doing different things for my health, one of which is taking the herb on regular basis. They really put you at whole different level than most plants.

My idea is you have these top herbs and it's not like there is an unlimited amount of these. There's a hundred in the Chinese medicine system. Then of course, there are other great herbal systems from around the world. Instead of focusing on the inferior herbs that may help with one thing or another… Why not focus on some of the best herbs in the world? That's my point of view, and that is what I have done with my herb company.

KALI: That's amazing! It's amazing to go beyond levels. For example, you could be on an airplane and everyone is coughing around you and you walk out, you are feeling fine, you feel great. You consciously know you have such a high immune system you don't even think about it.

LOGAN: I have no fear of being around sick people. I know they are not going to affect me because my immune system is at such a high level where it can fight off invaders. I have absolutely no problem. I can be around a person with the flu and it wont bother me.

KALI: Yeah that's a huge thing this time of year. During the holidays, we're constantly exposed to situations where you are closed in tight with others. It's cold outside and you know if someone has a cough you could 'catch' that. I would love to be at a level where nothing can touch me.

LOGAN: And so that's really the focus point with these herbs: its really health first and peak performance second. If you're taking drugs and some other herbs and supplements you can get some effects. But is it really going to be supporting your health in the long-term?

You know I'm after longevity and having a long run with the strength stuff. I want more than just being able to do these feats in my youth, my younger years. So it's important to me that my health really comes first and that is one of the biggest differences between taking herbs for these reasons versus taking drugs like Viagra.

KALI: Right because Viagra is just treating the symptoms temporarily. These herbs you can actually take and get the effects over the years. That's powerful. That's really powerful.

Having that type of control too - you don't have to be dependent on a doctor for your health, where you have to ask her for another prescription for Viagra. Because you take care of yourself when you take these herbs.

The biggest questions I get is, "are the herbs are going to work for different ages from 20's to 70's?" Is this going to work for the guys aged between 50's and 70's?

LOGAN: Yes, absolutely!

In fact, we just did a survey recently that found the majority of our customer-base is older males. These are the people who really need hormonal support. I think it's about time we actually talk about what these herbs are specifically.

One of the herbs carried by my company, that most people haven't heard about, is *pine pollen*. Pine pollen comes from the pine tree. If you are in some areas around the world, yellow dust —pollen — coats everyone's cars. This dust is actually a very potent herb. Every specie's pollen is different, so do NOT just go out and scrape it off your car.

The most interesting thing about pine pollen is that it's a phyto-androgen. Many people who have gotten into health and nutrition have heard of phyto-estrogens, which are compounds in things such as flax seeds, hops and soybeans that mimic estrogen in the human body. There is some controversy about phyto-estrogens – some of these can have good effects, but many of us are overloaded with estrogens. Estrogens are also in plastics, pesticides and other chemicals. Most people are getting way to much estrogen in their bodies.

Men do need a small amount of estrogen, but too much is going to result in having lower testosterone. Having a lower sex drive. Increased fat deposits around the abdominal area. You can have bitch tits. These are all consequences of having too much estrogen. [Picture: Estrogen dominant man.]

There are a few of these things in plant foods. Phyto-androgens such as those found in pine pollen is very rare. What you actually find in pine pollen are supports for testosterone, DHEA and a couple of other male sex hormones. A lot of herbs can help boost testosterone in different ways by having things such as zinc and other important minerals for testosterone balance. Pine pollen will actually be bio-available for humans to take.

KALI: That's amazing! I actually went out and did the whole saliva tests for my hormone levels.

I was estrogen dominant as a female. But with my male clients I've noticed estrogen dominance and if they are not taking things like pine pollen that are really powerful and natural and synergestic that can help over a long period of time... They really do get the weight around the abdomen. They get bitch tits. Interestingly, as men age, their estrogen levels increase. It's really important to do hormone balancing. I know right away just by looking if a man is estrogen-dominant because the physical signs are very apparent.

LOGAN: Yeah there's so many estrogens in our environment. We get these from things like plastics and chemicals. It's hard to avoid.

Pine pollen has these male sex hormones in them.

I was just talking about these superior herbs and when you take it in a powder form it's going to help to balance and regulate your hormones to some level. Is this going work us well as getting hormonal replacement where it's actually injected with testosterone? You know probably not but it is a first step.

Some people certainly need that. If you are an older man go to your doctor and talk about that. It can be something that works really great for you. But why not start something that is a lot cheaper, generally safer, and can be done over the longer term. If you start something a little earlier in your life you can get the benefits of regulating your hormones through taking something like this.

KALI: Exactly! The biggest problem I hear from men is: "why should I go see a doctor? Because you know I have to ask her repeatedly for Viagra or for testosterone injections and does my insurance pay for it? And a lot of people want to stay discreet. They don't want to go their doctor and tell him they have a problem. So this is where you could actually do a lot of self-help, self-supplementation of the pine pollen.

LOGAN: Yeah and we get a lots of great reports from our customer as far as benefits. You mentioned this we just recently put out a Morning-Wood guarantee.

KALI: Yeah! I mentioned that!!!

LOGAN: Let me talk a little bit about this. In doing research, we found that in China they take greater dosages than generally recommended of the pine pollen. In powdered form it's a bit different when you have it in a tincture or alcohol extract form. I'll talk about that in a minute. When you are taking the powder you can take a lot of it and its really going to help balance and regulate the hormones.

We came up with this guarantee based on our own experiments where you take the herb with three tablespoon of water at night. Then we can guarantee that you would wake up with morning wood. Now I can't guarantee that it will work for you, but this is something that we have found that works really well for many men.

So it's something worth trying out. I offer a satisfaction-guarantee, I just ask you to give it a couple uses to give the herbs a chance to work. Then there can be other things that are going on that would prevent it from working, but this is certainly something that would help in the vast majority of cases. If it doesn't work for you then we offer you one hundred percent of your money back – that is our 'morning wood' guarantee!

KALI: I have some of that in my cupboard – perhaps I should spike my boyfriend's drink. Hopefully he doesn't taste it.

LOGAN: Yeah, we get lots of reports from girlfriends who are very happy with the results from our herbs. Not just for themselves and others, and also for men who are spiking their girlfriend's drinks with these herbs as well. They boost libido in both sexes.

KALI: Yeah, okay no one heard that. I'm not going to go home and do that tonight. Logan knows my boyfriend.

We have a couple of questions and also let me ask you… Can people who have high blood pressure or diabetes take these herbs?

LOGAN: This something that you should know, just a legal disclaimer: you should absolutely talk your doctor about using herbs for their health-promoting effects. Like we talked about how it's not just like taking Viagra and all you get is just a boner.

There's a lot of nutrition in these herbs, and they can have many effects that may cause you to have to change the dosage of your medications.

We have reports from a few people that pine pollen helped get them off their blood pressure medications. This is something you should talk about to your doctor. Obviously you don't want to mess with your medications yourself. But the sad truth is most doctors wont have heard about these herbs. They will probably say no, that it will not help at all. But yeah we have received reports of the healthy effects pine pollen has with blood pressure and some others herb as well.

As far as diabetes, one of the herbs we have that helps is Shilajit. It is known to help regulate blood sugar levels. By taking these herbs you may need to alter the dosage of your medications because they really do help. Talk to your doctor.

KALI: You should talk to your doctor, and the interesting thing is your doctor probably will have no knowledge. What you should do is go to Logan's website or you can go online and start searching these herbs and print out the information and hand it to your doctor. Your doctor will be amazed. And you can even hand the herbs to your doctor and go, "hey try these out too." How can he make a judgment if he hasn't tried them himself? It really depends on what type of personality the doctor has. If he is an extreme allopath-Nazi than he is going to ignore you.

LOGAN: What we're trying to do more on the website now is actually back everything we say with scientific data. I've been quoting studies on all these different herbs. We're still going to go and add a bunch more. We're adding source material for all the different herbs on what they have been studied for and for their different benefits. Some of herbs have been studied about more than others. Most of the research comes from China, Japan and other countries because they have richer history on herbalism than we do here in United States.

So we're trying to make that information available so it stops the quackery and it's really backed by science. Why not try it for yourself? I can tell you the stories of people and the results of our clients and the reviews which are available on our website but try it for yourself. See if it works for you. That's the best test available: whether these things for you.

KALI: And that also goes back to dosage, what you are eating and how you exercise and the stress you have in your life. Earlier we talked about what biologically happens and what causes you to have weak/low erections. There are three things you really need take into consideration:

dosage, exercise, stress levels and what you are eating, the nutritional you taking in. What makes the herbs incredible is they go beyond this and act as form of super nutrition.

LOGAN: Absolutely right. In many ways they can take over the place of multivitamins or minerals. Pine Pollen is a complete protein, it has all the different essential amino acids, lots of vitamins and minerals, which includes zinc.

KALI: So lets go to the questions of the people who were listening to the Bliss Show. Here is the first one. Nick asks, **"Can any herb increase the penis size?"**

LOGAN: Yes thank you Nick...I'm not going to come out to say 'yes' but we have heard from couple of our customers that one of our herbs, the ant extract, has done that for them. Let me talk a little bit about the herb because it can seem like a weird thing when you first hear about it. This is a specific type of ant known as the Polyrhachis Ant that lives only in a mountainous region of China.

These ants are much larger than ants here in the United States. This herb is actually a more powerful Qi tonic than ginseng, which is thought of as a powerful Qi tonic herb itself.

Let me just say something about ginseng. Most people may have seen ginseng at a 7 Eleven or other convenience store. The products are often called a "Natural Energy Tonic." Most ginseng herb sold in the market is complete crap, as you really need to have mature ginseng in order to get the herb's true effects. But the ant extract has a lot of amazing things about it. First, it supplies ATP (Adenosine triphosphate, a co-enzyme used as an energy carrier in the cells of all known organisms) directly to your body. So it gives you a lot of energy. It's the highest source of zinc of anything on the planet.

Oysters have some zinc but Black Ant has even more zinc than oysters. As I mentioned before, zinc is a critical mineral for testosterone production. It is also needed for muscular contraction and for a whole bunch of things in the body. Most people are chronically deficient in zinc so that's the one benefits of Black Ant.

Oysters were a favorite of Cassanova – if this 'womanizer' had been Chinese, he would have used Black Ant instead.

Kali: Orgasm is a muscle contraction within the prostate gland. Now just imagine how powerful these orgasms are on black ant extract that acts to intensify contractions.

LOGAN: I personally maily use the herb for pre-workouts, but there are other uses. <u>These herbs can help increase the power of your orgasm as well</u>. Like I've said we have reports from some customers who actually had their penis get bigger from using this. This may not work for you but once again it is something you can try.

One story I like to tell is about a guy who was at work and took some of the ant extract on his lunch break. He started talking with some of the women, and they accused him of going home and getting a "quickie" just because he seemed a lot happier. His mood shift was just because of the Black Ant Extract. It was like the Black Ant Extract can give some sort of energy that women notice as well.

KALI: That is incredible. Imagine women turning around and smiling just because you have a sexual energy glow from taking the Black Ant Extract.

LOGAN: Yes. It's one of my favorite herbs of all. Like I've said, I've used it before doing my workouts and there's a lot of benefits for doing the Black Ant Extract. Including the nutritional content of the minerals, vitamins and also the energy vibrancy of the herb.

KALI: I have a question from Cecil and I think Cecil is not from United States. He asks, "Are these secret herbs approve by the Food And Drug Administration? Are there side effects? If these herbs are effective how come they have not been known?"

LOGAN: Okay. Thank you Cecil they are not approved by the FDA for any specific use. Their use is protected by the Dietary Supplement and Health Education Act, which is the law that keeps the big pharmaceutical companies from exterminating natural health suppliers. This means you can take them because they are not "drugs", they're merely food. That is a different way to think of it. If you desire to achieve radiant health, you appreciate the protection of the DSHEA.

Think of the food pyramid, the horribly flawed visual guide to eating. This was published by the US Department of Agriculture.

The superior herbs, if you had those on a daily basis then your health would be much better.

Speaking of the FDA, I would not trust them for all your health information. Their job is to approve drugs sold by the drug companies. The drug industry has a lot of influence at the FDA. They put drugs that have very bad side effects, that kill people and often times they take years for it to come to light to pull it off the market. The FDA surely does some good protecting you but surely it is not wise to look to it for all your health information. As for why most people don't know about these herbs? It's just because most people don't because stuff like the FDA say, "supplements are just worthless." "It's going to hurt you when they're pumping out drugs that definitely proven to cause problems."

KALI: Exactly! Most of the board members on the FDA are also board members of MONSANTO. Monsanto already dominates America's food chain with its genetically modified seeds. Now it has targeted milk production. Just as frightening as the corporation's tactics – ruthless legal battles against small farmers – is its decades-long history of toxic contamination.

It's really important to know who and where you are getting your information from and if they have another agenda. The FDA is there to plant suggestions in your mind that you are helpless and that you can't do anything for yourself. I mean come on it's all about money and making us docile. They're not here to help us.

LOGAN: Exactly.

KALI: Okay next question. Mike asks, "Does any herb help with premature ejaculation?"

LOGAN: Interesting question. I have experienced from myself longer lasting stamina by taking herbs like the Black Ant Extract and Shilajit. I have also heard this from numerous customers, so that could help in that regard. I have a story: one guy was taking Shilajit and he seemed to keep going even after ejaculating. He remained hard and kept going. I personally heard that from of one of my customer's girlfriends. She was very, very happy about it.

Get The Herbs Here

http://www.kaliblissshow.com/herbs

Recommended Resources

Sexual Energy Healing For Men:

http://www.EnergyViagra.com

Hypnosis For Sex:

http://www.HypnosisForSex.com

KALI: That's a great side effect!

It's interesting because in the Kama Sutra there's actually writing about secrets herbs. They are written in a kind of a code; it's not that transparent in the English translations. The Kama Sutra talks about a herb that could provide double ejaculatory orgasms and the hardness factor to please a harem. The writings in the Kama Sutra are very old, and no one has any real identification of what the herb is now.

I wonder now if Shilajit is the herb talked about in the Kama Sutra that helps men keep on going.

LOGAN: I wouldn't be surprised - Shilajit comes from India. Yeah its one of the top anti-aging herbs. Its nickname "the destroyer of weakness," or "the conqueror of mountains". Another nickname is "Indian Viagra." It's a very potent herb and has far-reaching effects.

These herbs are very health supporting. You may be taking them for enhanced sexual function but you'll notice a lot of other benefits. The side effects are beneficial. You might begin to notice you have a lot of energy. A lot of people notice they have a lot less joint pain. They have noticed their digestion and nervous system improved. They have noticed their immune system increasing. You are going to see beneficial side effects with herbs like these.

KALI: Luis asks, "Are the herbs better than L-Argenine for hard, lasting erections?

LOGAN: It's hard to say, for some people because the body is very complex. L-Argenine may be exactly what they need in order to get benefits. Like I described the nitric oxide, some herbs have L-Argenine in them. They can help boost nitric oxide and for some people other herbs are better.

Like you were saying about L-Argenine Kali, some people were taking massive amounts of it. This is a bit more than the body can handle. It is not something you want to do all the time. So like I said, experiment on yourself to find what works for you. You can even combine the two to see what happens.

KALI: L-Argenine is the precursor to synthesize into nitric oxide and they (the FDA) say you literally need only 5 grams just to have daily value consumption of L-Argenine. Well the thing is, seven of my clients went and tested and they were all they way up to 25grams a day to have the sexual effects.

LOGAN: There's one thing I can say about that L-Argenine – it has an effect, but what else is there in order for you to start producing the nitric oxide? Nothing in our body really works alone. What about co-factors used in the production?

KALI: Yes, are you getting the nutrients to break down the L-Argenine. Taking L-Argenine alone may not have the same effect as it would with the other nutrients that help with its process over into nitric oxide.

LOGAN: When you have whole foods and herbs, those co-factors tend to be there. Generally, individual supplements can definitely be great, but they tend to be imbalanced. You really have to play with it. One thing might work better for one person and another might work another person. So these are something you really want to experiment with on yourself.

HOW TO TAKE IT

KALI: Let me tell you about what I do in the morning. I go into the kitchen and I put the tap on because we live here in the backwards where the waters is crystal clear. There are no additives or fluoride in our water. I put the tap on to let the water warm up. I go to my cabinet and pull out my Black Ant Extract and Pine pollen. I get my other supplements and I mix them in a glass with warm water. I take that. It's the first thing I take in the morning and I let it sit for a half an hour for it to digest completely in an empty stomach.

I've had some serious effects from this. Again its about how you take it.

When you take it. The dosage.

And also what you are taking it with are co-factors your body uses to break it down. This makes for even more powerful and potent experience with the herbs.

Sometimes it is about getting up in morning and having that intense Superfood cocktail. Let it sit, let it digest. Popping a pill after you have eaten a burger isn't going to help. There is a process to having it work.

LOGAN: Absolutely!!! You can take them in different ways. Some herbs, for some people taking them with food may be better but like you, I like taking the herbs on an empty stomach. For me, this way I think the herbs' effects are better.

Let me talk about how much you are going to feel from these herbs. If you take these herbs in a small dose you may not notice right away. It's not going to be 'instant' like Viagra. To get the Viagra-effect it may end up taking a couple of weeks to get your sexual hormone levels increased naturally. However there *is* something in the Black Ant Extract that people feel right away but it's not like a drug effect. Understand it is subtle, meaning it may take time depending on where you are at with your health.

KALI: Yes it really important to know what dosage to take and how to take it.

We have more questions.

Mike from Los Angeles purchased the pine pollen. He wants to know how much he should take and how long he should take it for. He is in his late 50's and is a little overweight, but he exercises for an hour 5 days a week. He's in a high stress job. Could you give him a little hint about what he should take and how long he should take it for him to get the effects? Thank you.

HOW MUCH TO TAKE

LOGAN: Okay so what we recommend for the starting point for people is 1/2 to 1 teaspoon a day twice a day. That can be a good start. In fact, for many people they're going to feel the results after taking that. If you were to contrast the Morning Wood Guarantee we say take 3 tablespoons, heaping tablespoons, and to do that at night before you go to bed. These herbs you can definitely play with the dosages. You have to find out what works well for you. In older males typically as you aged your hormone levels declined. The male sex hormones are going down so a lot of people find they can get the benefits with very minimal dosage.

Now if you want more testosterone and hormonal effects what you can do with the pine pollen is get an alcohol extract of it or create your own. We actually have a video and details on our website on how to do that.

When you are using the alcohol extract with pine pollen it's going to draw out those hormones. You will notice how they are going to be much more bio-available in your body when you just take it sublingually, under the tongue. What happens with the hormones, when you ingest a powder they don't get absorbed easily into the body. It still has a balancing and regulating effect, but hormones can be boosted more with the alcohol form.

So that's something you can play with as well. If you do that, I've noticed that for myself, I get a hormonal boost when I take it in that form.

This is better for older men. This is something that women don't want to do because it has the anabolic effects in the tinctured form. The powdered form is safer. Even children can take the powder but generally only men 30 years or older should really experiment with tinctured alcohol forms.

KALI: Let me ask you this, if they take it sublingually under the tongue it will go right into the bloodstream? That's fast acting.

LOGAN: That will be absorbed into the bloodstream, which is why it works with the tinctured form rather than powder. Its effects are little bit different, hormones go right in with that but if you take them in the stomach they to tend to end up absorbing into the body.

KALI: So that's really fast and an easy way to get that into you.

LOGAN: I want to have this done. We haven't done it yet but in the future we probably will be funding people and giving pine pollen and then making them get blood work before and after. This will really show the hormonal effects. But that is something we don't have right now but it's coming the future.

KALI: Here is another question for you. Dr. Doug from Michigan asks, "Is it used in China by Traditional Chinese Medicine Practitioners? Is it used by Tibetan Monks? How is it different than the thousand of herbs I get emails about?"

LOGAN: These herbs were something that was use by mystics and people who lived high up on the mountains, and the Shaolin Monks. These herbs were a part of their diet. With the idea of monks that had sort of super powers that really were hidden away and there are a whole bunch of legends. The idea is they removed themselves more and more off food, and they just consumed these herbs as their food. They would make a stew from different roots and herbs. Their food supply was a tonic of really powerful herbs.

A lot of legends about that and a long history. If you go to the Chinese temples you will see the artwork on the Reshi mushrooms, which is one of the most well-known and highest regarded of these tonic herbs out there. These herbs were really to increase your "Shen" which is sort of the Chinese idea of spirit. Developing "Shen" is important for people that are meditating to achieve enlightenment. There are all kind of different stories that go back a long, long time ago.

KALI: It's amazing how they actually made these herbs a cornerstone of their diet, of what they were consuming. Then they used this level of consumption to achieve a higher level of enlightenment. They developed the physical body by ingesting herbs they knew would get them to that level.

LOGAN: Unfortunately now most of our food supply has many additives that heighten the taste of everything. We've lost the ability to taste real food. If you go deep within these herbs you can actually understand and feel the effects of the different herbs. You begin to notice the effects as they enter the energetic meridians of the body.

If you pay attention and work on these herbs you actually can begin to feel the effects moving across your meridians as you take them. You can go definitely very far into processing the herbs on different levels of awareness.

KALI: So you can imagine a meditation based on the meridians. For those that know about acupuncture, there are 14 pathways on the human body and they're fixed pathways that have emotional components. The meridians provide energy to different organ groups.

LOGAN: Many people have found that these herbs are a gateway into a more spiritual life. It helps you get in more touch with yourself and the universe. The herbs help open up these channels. You start to take one, and it leads you to another one. So it can be a good place to start.

There are a lot of people in my field who are doing strength training. If you do the training right, you get great results. The herbs to me, are one of my secret weapons they don't have or know anything about for strength training.

I guess they're not so secret now that I have revealed them, but they're not something that everybody does. I find that the herbs enhance all the results that I can get by bringing all those things together. Just like when we were talking about peak performance.

KALI: Bring it all together.

I have another question this question is from BJ, "What does Logan think about during sex?"

LOGAN: Okay… I focus on the present, on my partner and I stay in the moment.

KALI: The present – you try being on your present, being present on your physical body, just like we talk on meditation, you can really start to feel a vibration, a tingling sensation. But it does take learning how to get there, in the moment.

You actually have to train the mind and train the body. Most people never are properly trained when it comes to sex. They are physically dissociated from their bodies.

LOGAN: I don't think about baseball so that I can last longer.

KALI: Here's the thing, most women will be looking at the ceiling, right?! Here's the thing - you want her feel the urge, you want her to feel the vibrations, you want her to feel the sensations and the circulation amplified by the herbs that pulsate through your penis. You also want to be there, feel her physical body next to you in the present where time slows down.

LOGAN: I totally agree.

KALI: Logan I have another question. Can you explain more about herbs that give men sexual effects that are long lasting.

LOGAN: Absolutely. I would definitely experiment with all the herbs that I talked about: the Pine Pollens, Shilajit, and another one I want to mention is He Shou Wu. This is another top herb in tonic Chinese Herbalism.

A legend to this herb, He Shou Wu actually means Mr. Wu's hairy back or something along those lines. I've heard different translations, but there was man whom at age 58 and was never married because he was impotent. He had lots of problems with impotency.

So at the age of 58 one day he got drunk in the forest and fell asleep. He had a dream where he noticed roots that appeared to be making love. When he woke up he noticed these roots were right next to him. So he dug them up and made it into a tonic he would consume.

Within a short period of time he noticed a new energy flowing in his body. He began to feel stimulated and could hardly contain his sexual drive. He continued taking He Shou Wu for years and he also noticed that his grey hair turned black and he fathered many children. The legend says he lived until he was 160 years old, and fathered 19 sons and daughters. As I said earlier this was starting at the age of 58.
Legends can be exaggerated a bit but there's some truth to this. These herbs are quite powerful and we actually put together a formula combining these things we talked about today. It's called the Phoenix formula. The Phoenix is the mythical fire bird comes from the ashes and burns again. That's how the idea of this powerful formula came to be. It's really supporting to having your sex life again.

Get The Herbs Here

http://www.kaliblissshow.com/herbs

Recommended Resources

Sexual Energy Healing For Men:

http://www.EnergyViagra.com

Hypnosis For Sex:

http://www.HypnosisForSex.com

www.ingramcontent.com/pod-product-compliance
Lightning Source LLC
Chambersburg PA
CBHW050924290526
45792CB00002B/871